The Code of Wellbeing

A Path to Complete Health and Well-Being

BY

Winifred C. Brandon

DISCLAIMER

This information is not meant to replace medical advice and treatment, or to offer medical advice. It is highly recommended that readers seek the advice of a licensed medical practitioner before treating any medical concerns. In addition to any loss, damage, or injury caused or claimed to be caused directly or indirectly by any information, action, or application of any food or food source discussed in this book, the author and publisher disclaim all liability and responsibility for any misinterpretation or misuse of the information contained in this book. No warranties are made by the author or publisher with regard to this basic information. The purpose of this information is not to identify, treat, or eliminate any illness.

INTRODUCTION

Maintaining a nutritious diet throughout your life can help ward against several non-communicable diseases (NCDs) and ailments, as well as malnutrition in all its manifestations. Nonetheless, a change in dietary habits has been brought about by a rise in the manufacturing of processed foods, fast urbanization, and altered lifestyles. These days, a lot of people don't eat enough fruit, vegetables, or other dietary fiber-rich foods like whole grains. Instead, they eat more meals high in fats, sugars that aren't processed, salt, and potassium.

A varied, balanced, and healthful diet's precise composition will differ based on an individual's attributes (such as age, gender, lifestyle, and level of physical activity), the cultural setting, the foods that are readily available in the area, and dietary habits. Still, there are certain fundamental ideas about what makes a healthy diet.

HEALTHY DIETS

A diet that preserves or enhances general health is considered healthy. The body gets its basic nutrition from a balanced diet, which includes enough fiber, water, macronutrients like protein, micronutrients like vitamins, and dietary energy.

Fruits, vegetables, and whole grains can all be found in a healthy diet, along with little to no ultra-processed food and beverages with added sugar. A range of foods, both plant- and animal-based, can provide the requirements for a healthy diet; however, vegans require additional sources of vitamin B12.

For adults, a healthy diet consists of the following: Fruits and vegetables, whole grains, nuts, legumes (such beans and lentils), and unprocessed maize, millet, oats, and wheat

5 servings, or at least 400 g, of fruit and vegetables each day; do not include potatoes, sweet potatoes, cassava, or other starchy roots.

Less than 10 percent of total energy intake comes from free sugar, which is equal to 50 grams, or roughly 12 level teaspoons, for an individual with a healthy body weight who consumes 2000 calories a day. For further health benefits, the amount should ideally be less than 5 percent of total energy intake. All added sugars to food or beverages, whether by the producer, chef, or customer, as well as sugars found naturally in honey, syrups, fruit juices, and fruit juice concentrates, are considered free sugars. Less than 30 percent of calories come from fat. Unsaturated fats, which are present in fish, avocado, and nuts as well as sunflower, soybean, canola, and olive oils, are better than saturated fats, which are present in fatty meat, butter, palm and coconut oil, cream, cheese, ghee, and lard, as well as trans fats of all kinds, which include both ruminant and industrially produced trans fats, which are present in meat and dairy products from ruminant animals like cows, sheep, goats, and camels, as well as pre-packaged snacks and foods like frozen pizza, pies, biscuits, wafers, and cooking oils and spreads. Saturated fat consumption should be limited to less than 10% of total energy intake, while trans-fat consumption should be limited to less than 1%. Specifically, trans-fats generated industrially are not a component of a healthy diet and are to be avoided. Approximately one teaspoon's worth, or less than five grams, of salt daily. Salt should be iodize.

For babies and young kids

Optimal diet during a child's first two years of life promotes healthy growth and enhances cognitive development. Additionally, it lowers the chance of gaining weight or becoming obese and eventually getting NCDs.

The guidelines for a nutritious diet for babies and kids are the same as those for adults, but they should also include the following things:

A baby should only be nursed for the first six months of its life.

Breastfeeding should be continued for infants until they are two years old and older.

Breast milk should be supplemented with a range of sufficient, secure, and nutrient-dense foods starting at six months of age. Complementary foods shouldn't have sugar or salt added to them.

Some suggestions

World Health Organization

The World Health Organization (WHO) suggests the following five measures for both people and populations:

Eating about equal to your body's calorie needs will help you maintain a healthy weight.

30% of total calories should come from fats, with unsaturated fats being preferred over saturated fats. Skip the trans-fats.

Consume 400 grams or more of fruits and vegetables per day (sweet potatoes, cassava, potatoes, and other starchy roots excluded). Legumes (such as beans and lentils), whole grains, and nuts are other components of a balanced diet. Consume no more than as little simple sugar as possible.

10% of total calories (less than 5% of calories, or 25 grams, would be even better).

Make sure all salt is iodized and limit your intake of salt and sodium. Lowering daily salt intake to less than 5 grams can lower the risk of cardiovascular disease.

According to the WHO, 2.8% of fatalities globally are attributable to a lack of fruits and vegetables.

The WHO also suggests the following other:

Ensuring that the meals selected contain enough of a given vitamin and mineral

Avoiding compounds that are immediately carcinogenic (benzene) and toxic (heavy metals).

A diet low in saturated fats and high in polyunsaturated fats can lower the incidence of diabetes and coronary artery disease. Avoiding items infected with human pathogens (such as E. Coli and tapeworm eggs).

American Institute for Cancer Research; American Heart Association; World Cancer Research Fund

A diet high in whole grains, legumes, and non-starchy fruits and vegetables is advised by the American Heart Association, World Cancer Research Fund, and American Institute for Cancer Research. A diverse array of non-starchy fruits and vegetables, including red, green, yellow, white, purple, and orange, are part of this nutritious diet.

The guidelines mention that cruciferous vegetables like cauliflower, allium crops like garlic, and cooked tomatoes in oil may offer some cancer-prevention benefits. The low energy density of this nutritious meal may help prevent weight gain and related illnesses. Finally, cutting back on energy-dense meals like "fast foods" and red meat as well as avoiding processed meats will all help you live a longer and healthier life. Overall, scientists and decision-makers in the medical field determine that eating a balanced diet can lower the risk of cancer and chronic illnesses.

Children should limit their daily intake of added sugar to 25 grams or less (100 calories). Additional guidelines suggest limiting sugar intake for children under two years old and consuming no more than one soft drink each week. In order to minimize the risk of cardiovascular disease, it is now advised to increase intake of monounsaturated and polyunsaturated fats while decreasing consumption of saturated fats. As of 2018, decreasing overall fat consumption is no longer suggested.

Advantages of a nutritious diet

Nutrient-dense foods from all of the major food groups, such as lean proteins, whole grains, healthy fats, and a variety of colored fruits and vegetables, are usually found in a balanced diet. Trans-fats, added salt, and sugar-containing meals should be swapped out for healthier alternatives as part of a healthy eating regimen.

Maintaining a nutritious diet can prevent disease, strengthen bones, shield the heart, and improve mood, among many other advantages.

10 advantages of a nutritious diet and the supporting data

Heart wellness

As stated by the Centers for Disease Control

Heart disease is the top cause of mortality for adults in the US, according to the Centers for Disease Control and Prevention (CDC).

Nearly half of American adults suffer from a cardiovascular illness of some kind, according to the American Heart Association (AHA).

In the United States, hypertension, or high blood pressure, is becoming a bigger problem. A heart attack, heart failure, or stroke may result from the illness. Changes in lifestyle, such as upping physical activity and eating a healthy diet, may be able to avoid up to 80% of early diagnoses of heart disease and stroke. Foods have the power to lower blood pressure and maintain cardiac health.

There are lots of heart-healthy foods in the Dietary Approaches to Stop Hypertension (DASH) diet. Consuming an abundance of fruits, vegetables, and whole grains is advised by the program.

Selecting fish, poultry, legumes, nuts, vegan or low-fat dairy products, and vegetable oils

Restricting consumption of foods high in trans and saturated fats, such as full-fat dairy and fatty meats

Reducing the amount of foods and beverages with added sugars

Limiting daily sodium consumption to less than 2,300 mg, preferably 1,500 mg, and boosting potassium, magnesium, and calcium intake

Consuming foods high in fiber is also essential for maintaining heart health.

According to the American Heart Association, eating dietary fiber decreases blood cholesterol and reduces the risk of obesity, type 2 diabetes, heart disease, and stroke. The connection between trans-fats and heart-related conditions such coronary heart disease has long been acknowledged by the medical community.

Reducing specific fat types can also help heart health. For example, cutting out trans-fats lowers LDL (low-density lipoprotein) cholesterol levels. This kind of cholesterol raises the risk of heart attacks and strokes by causing plaque to build up in the arteries.

Additionally, lowering blood pressure can improve heart health. The majority of adults may accomplish this by consuming no more than 1,500 mg of salt per day.

Many processed and quick foods are seasoned with salt by food makers; those who want to reduce their blood pressure should stay away from these items.

Lower chance of cancer

By shielding their cells from harm, meals high in antioxidants can help lower a person's chance of getting cancer.

Free radicals raise the body's risk of cancer, but antioxidants assist the body rid itself of them, reducing the chance of developing the illness.

Numerous phytochemicals, such as beta carotene, lycopene, and vitamins A, C, and E, are present in fruits, vegetables, nuts, and legumes and work as antioxidants.

Studies conducted in labs and on animals have shown a connection between specific antioxidants and a lower risk of cancer-related free radical damage. Doctors warn against utilizing these dietary supplements without first consulting them because human research have yielded conflicting results.

Antioxidant-rich foods include;

Raspberries and blueberries, among other berries.

Rich, dark greens

Carrots and squash

Fruits and nuts

Obesity may worsen a person's chances of getting cancer as well as raise that risk. Keeping a healthy weight may help lower these risks.

A fruit-rich diet was found to lower the risk of upper gastrointestinal tract malignancies in a 2014 study.

Additionally, they discovered that a diet high in fruits, vegetables, and fiber decreased the risk of colorectal cancer and that a diet high in fiber decreased the risk of liver cancer.

Happier disposition

There is evidence to support the notion that nutrition and mood are closely related. Researchers discovered in 2016 that individuals with obesity who are otherwise healthy may have more symptoms of weariness and sadness while following a diet high in glycemic load.

Numerous refined carbs, including those in soft drinks, cakes, biscuits, and white bread, are part of a diet high in glycemic load. Whole grains, vegetables, and fruit all have a lower glycemic load.

Additionally, recent studies have revealed that a person's diet can influence immunological response, gut microbiome, and blood glucose levels—all of which have an impact on mood. Additionally, the researchers discovered a potential connection between improved mental health and healthier diets like the Mediterranean diet. On the other hand, diets heavy in processed, high-fat, and red meat items have the opposite effect.

It is significant to remember that the researchers emphasized the need for more investigation into the processes underlying the relationship between diet and mental health. Speaking with a physician or mental health specialist could be beneficial for someone who thinks they may be experiencing depressive symptoms.

Better digestive health

Numerous naturally occurring bacteria that are vital to digestion and metabolism reside in the colon. Additionally, some bacterial strains generate vitamins B and K, which are good for the colon. They might also aid in the battle against dangerous viruses and germs. A high-fiber diet may help reduce gastrointestinal irritation. Prebiotics and probiotics from a diet high in fiber vegetables, fruits, legumes, and whole grains may help promote the growth of healthy bacteria in the colon.

Probiotic-rich fermented foods include yogurt and sauerkraut, miso Kefir

Prebiotics have the potential to alleviate a variety of digestive problems, such as the symptoms of irritable bowel syndrome (IBS).

Improved memory

Maintaining brain health and cognition may be aided by a nutritious diet.

Nevertheless, further thorough investigation is required.

Nutrients and meals that guard against dementia and cognitive decline were found in a 2015 study. The following were considered to be advantageous by the researchers;

Nutrients C, D, and E

The fatty acids omega-3

Polyphenols and Flavonoids

Fish

Numerous of these nutrients are included in the Mediterranean diet, among other diets.

Loss of weight Reducing the chance of long-term health problems can be achieved by maintaining a moderate weight.

An individual who is obese or overweight may be more susceptible to various illnesses, such as;

Ischemic heart disease

Diabetes type 2

Arthritic bones

Headache

Blood pressure

A few mental health issues

Certain cancers

Compared to most processed foods, a large number of nutrient-dense foods, such as fruits, vegetables, and beans, have lesser calories. Without counting calories, someone can keep below their daily limit by eating a balanced diet.

Control of diabetes

A person with diabetes may benefit from a nutritious diet;

Control their glycemic levels

Maintain goal ranges for their blood pressure and cholesterol.

Avoid or postpone diabetes-related consequences

Keep your weight in check.

Limiting the amount of added sugar and salt in their diet is crucial for diabetics. Avoiding fried foods that are high in trans and saturated fats should also be an option.

Wholesome teeth and bones

Strong bones and teeth require a diet high in calcium and magnesium. Osteoporosis and other bone problems can be avoided later in life by maintaining good bone health.

Foods high in calcium include;

Dairy products

Lettuce

Green beans

Fish in a can with bones

Food makers frequently add calcium fortification to cereals, tofu, and plant-based milk. Many foods are high in magnesium, and some of the greatest ones are as follows:

Green leafy vegetables

Nuts

Seeds

Whole grains

Achieving improved sleep

Sleep apnea is one of the many conditions that might interfere with sleep cycles. When a disorder persistently obstructs the airways during sleep, it results in sleep apnea. Alcohol consumption and obesity are risk factors.

Reducing alcohol and caffeine use may aid in achieving peaceful sleep for everyone, with or without sleep apnea.

The future generation's health

Kids pick up most health-related habits from the people in their lives, so parents who set an example of eating well and exercising frequently likely to instill similar habits in their children.

Dining in may be beneficial as well. Researchers discovered in 2018 that kids who regularly ate meals with their family ate less sugary foods and more veggies than their peers, who ate at home less frequently.

Healthy eating guide/the nutrition source

Whether your meals are taken at the table or packed in a lunchbox, follow the Healthy Eating advice to prepare nutritious, well-balanced meals.

Developing a Well-Balanced Diet

Use ½ of your plate for fruits and vegetables to make up the majority of your meal.

Strive for color and diversity, and keep in mind that due to their detrimental effects on blood sugar, potatoes are not considered vegetables on the Healthy Eating Plate.

Aim for 25% of your plate to be made up of whole grains.

Compared to refined grains like white bread and white rice, whole and intact grains including whole wheat, barley, wheat berries, quinoa, oats, brown rice, and dishes produced from them like whole wheat pasta, have a lessening influence on insulin and blood sugar.

Protein power: one-half of your dish.

Nuts, beans, chicken, and fish are all wholesome, adaptable protein choices that go nicely with veggies on a platter or blended into salads. Cut back on red meat and stay away from processed meats like sausage and bacon.

Use healthy plant oils sparingly.

Avoid partly hydrogenated oils, which contain harmful trans-fats, and opt instead for nutritious vegetable oils like olive, canola, soy, maize, sunflower, peanut, and others. Keep in mind that "healthy" does not equate to low-fat.

Drink tea, coffee, or water.

Steer clear of sugar-filled beverages. Consume no more than one or two servings of milk or dairy products per day, and only one small glass of juice.

The type of carbohydrate in the diet is more important than the amount of carbohydrate in the diet, because some sources of carbohydrate—like vegetables (other than potatoes), fruits, whole grains, and beans are healthier than others.

This Healthy Eating guide also advises that you avoid sugary beverages, a major source of calories—usually with little nutritional value and use healthy oils.

Nutrients

Chemicals known as nutrients are present in all living organisms on Earth. They are essential to the survival of all living things, including humans, animals, and plants. In order to provide energy for living things, nutrients aid in the breakdown of food. They are utilized in every bodily function of an organism.

Nutrition and diet play a major role in your general health and well-being. Making sure your diet is full of nutrient-dense meals can provide you energy, maintain your body in optimal functioning condition, and aid in the healing process after different kinds of physical exercise and injury.

Six necessary nutrients and the reasons your body needs them.

Even in tiny doses, six fundamental nutrients can promote and maintain your health. You can make sure you're getting enough of each on a regular basis by eating a balanced diet.

Compounds that the body cannot produce, or cannot produce sufficiently, are known as essential nutrients. The World Health Organization states that these nutrients, which are essential for growth, health, and the prevention of disease, must come from food.

There are two types of nutrients that are considered essential: macronutrients and micronutrients.

The main nutritional components of your diet, protein, carbs, and fat, which provide your body energy, are macronutrients, which you eat in big quantities.

Micronutrients such as vitamins and minerals are highly concentrated in little amounts. Essential macronutrients and micronutrients fall into six major categories. There exist as;

Water, Protein, Carbohydrate, Fats, Vitamins, and Minerals

Protein

Protein is popular right now, and not just among athletes. But there's a legitimate reason for all the excitement. It takes protein to be healthy.

The building blocks of the body are found in protein, and not simply in muscle. Protein is present in every cell, including skin, hair, and bones.

Protein makes up a whopping 16 percent of the average person's body weight. Protein is mostly needed for bodily upkeep, growth, and health.

Protein makes up all of your hormones, antibodies, and other vital components. The body doesn't use protein as fuel unless absolutely required.

Different amino acids make up proteins. Although the body is able to produce some amino acids, food is the only source of several essential amino acids. Your body needs various kinds of amino acids to operate correctly.

Fortunately, you do not have to consume every amino acid at once. Complete proteins can be produced by your body from the foods you eat throughout the day.

Carbohydrate

A body that is healthy needs carbohydrates. Your body uses carbs as fuel, especially the brain and central nervous system, to fend off sickness. You should consume 45 to 65 percent of your daily calories as carbohydrates.

Fats

Although fats have a bad reputation, new research has demonstrated the importance of good fats in a balanced diet. Many bodily processes, including the absorption of vitamins and minerals, blood coagulation, cell division, and muscular contraction, are supported by lipids.

Although fat contains a lot of calories, your body needs those calories as fuel.

The World Health Organization advises limiting the amount of fat in your diet to less than 30% of total calories, whereas the Dietary Guidelines for Americans propose 20 to 35 percent.

By including healthy fats in your diet, you can lower your risk of heart disease and type 2 diabetes, balance your blood sugar, and enhance your cognitive function. They may reduce your chances of arthritis, cancer, and Alzheimer's disease. They are also potent anti-inflammatories.

Vitamin

Vitamins are essential for maintaining health and preventing illness. These micronutrients are necessary for the body to support its operations. The body needs 13 key vitamins, including vitamins A, C, B6, and D, in order to function correctly. Every vitamin has a crucial function in the body, and deficiency can lead to illnesses and other health issues. Many important vitamins are not sufficiently consumed by many Americans. Vitamins are necessary for strong bones, skin, and eyesight.

Vitamins are potent antioxidants that may reduce the incidence of prostate and lung cancer. Vitamins that support the immune system and aid in healing the body include vitamin C.

Minerals

Similar to vitamins, minerals aid in the body's support. They are necessary for a variety of bodily processes, such as maintaining healthy teeth and bones, controlling metabolism, and maintaining adequate hydration. The most prevalent minerals are zinc, iron, and calcium.

Calcium not only helps build stronger bones but also facilitates the passage of nerve signals, normal blood pressure, and the contraction and relaxation of muscles. Zinc strengthens your immune system and promotes wound healing, while iron helps your body produce hormones and red blood cells.

Water

Food can be skipped for weeks at a time, but water can only be gone for a few days at most. Water is essential to all of your body's systems. It's also the primary component of who you are. Water makes up about 62% of your body weight. Water elevates your mood and cognitive performance. It functions in the body as a lubricant and a shock absorber. In addition, it aids in toxin removal, nutrient delivery to cells, bodily hydration, and constipation avoidance.

Even slight dehydration can cause fatigue and negatively impact your focus and physical abilities.

The best method to obtain adequate amounts of these six vital nutrients, as well as the significant category of phytonutrients—the healthy compounds found in vibrant plants that fend against disease—is to eat a diversified diet full of fruits, vegetables, whole grains, and lean proteins and fats. Your body needs certain macronutrients and micronutrients in order to function properly and be healthy.

Junk foods

Food that has no dietary fiber, protein, vitamins, minerals, or other essential types of nutritional value but is very pleasant due to its high calorie content from sugar, fat, and/or sodium is referred to as "junk food." Although it is quick and simple to eat, it is also known as unhealthy foods.

Obesity is on the rise globally, increasing the risk of chronic illnesses including diabetes and heart disease. Although junk food can lead to obesity, our fast-paced lifestyles have made it a part of our daily existence. When you balance sports, school, and spending time with friends and family, life can get quite busy! Junk food firms have largely replaced cooking and eating healthful homemade meals since their products are tasty, handy, and reasonably priced. Fast food items such as burgers, fried chicken, and pizza, packaged foods like chips, biscuits, and ice cream, sugar-sweetened drinks like soda, fatty meats like bacon, sugary cereals, and frozen ready meals like lasagne are all considered junk food. These foods are usually highly processed, which means that several processes were taken to make the dish with the intention of making it pleasant and simple to overindulge in. Regretfully, junk food has a lot of calories and energy but not enough of the essential nutrients—like proteins, vitamins, minerals, and fiber—that our bodies require to grow and stay healthy. It's troubling that the majority of teenagers between the ages of 14 and 18 obtain more than 40% of their daily energy from these kinds of meals. Foods that are "not needed to meet nutrient requirements and do not belong to the five food groups" are referred to as junk food or discretionary foods. Grain and cereal combinations, fruits, vegetables and legumes, dairy products and substitutes, and meat and meat substitutes make up these five food groups.

Junk food firms frequently target young people with their devious advertising strategies, featuring our idols and icons endorsing junk food.

Junk food's effects on health

Food is composed of three main nutrients: lipids, proteins, and carbs. Food also contains vitamins and minerals that aid in growth, development, and overall health. It's critical that we have the right nourishment during our adolescent years. On the other hand, junk food contains large amounts of proteins, lipids, and carbs that the body absorbs very quickly.

Let's use eating a hamburger as an example. Proteins and fats from the beef patties, carbs from the bun, and fats from the cheese and sauce are the usual components of a burger. A fast-food chain burger typically provides 36–

40% of your daily energy requirements, not including any chips or beverages that may be taken with it. The body needs a lot of time to process this much of food.

The bread provides the majority of a burger's carbohydrates, but the beef patty provides the majority of its protein. There's a lot of fat in the cheese and sauce. For teenage boys between the ages of 12 and 15, a single burger can account for 36% of their daily energy consumption, while for teenage girls between the ages of 12 and 15, it can account for 40%.

After consuming rich, heavy foods like a burger, unpleasant symptoms like fatigue, restless nights, and even hunger can appear several hours to days later. Junk food may cause a decrease in energy levels rather than an increase in energy. People who consume sugar, a form of carbohydrate, feel happier, more energized, and more positive for a brief period of time until their bodies use it as fuel. However, because refined sugar is readily absorbed by the body, it causes a rapid drop in blood sugar levels. Refined sugar is the kind of sugar typically found in junk food. This may result in fatigue and cravings.

The Long-Term Effects of Junk Foods

There may be a number of long-term effects on health if we consume primarily junk food for numerous weeks, months, or years. For instance, there is a substantial correlation between high blood levels of bad cholesterol, which may indicate heart disease, and heavy consumption of saturated fats. Reputable studies have shown that young people with lower overall cholesterol levels eat relatively small amounts of saturated fat.

Regular junk food consumption also raises the risk of diseases like hypertension and stroke, which are defined as high blood pressure and brain damage from reduced blood supply that denies the brain oxygen and nutrients it needs to survive. These conditions are brought on by the high cholesterol and salt content of junk food, as well as the release of dopamine, the "happy hormone," which makes us feel good after eating it and makes us want more junk food to experience the same happy feeling again. Long-term consequences of junk food consumption also include tooth decay and constipation. Soft drinks, for example, have high levels of acid and sugar that can erode the tooth enamel's protective layer, leading to tooth disease. Junk food is usually poor in fiber as well, which over time can be detrimental to gut health. Our feces mostly consist of fiber, and it can be difficult to poop without it!

Junk food can cause short-term symptoms like fatigue, bloating, and difficulty concentrating. Junk food consumption over time might result in bad bowel habits and teeth damage. Junk food consumption can also contribute to obesity and related conditions like heart disease. The costs and health consequences of consuming junk food on a regular basis over an extended period of time rise.

Effects of fast food on eight bodily parts

It may happen more frequently than some of us would want to acknowledge—pulling into your favorite fast-food restaurant or utilizing the drive-through. On any given day between 2013 and 2016, 36.6% of American adults consumed fast food. From 2015 to 2018, 36.3% of children and adolescents ate fast food on any given day. This percentage was almost the same.

While the occasional fast food meal is harmless, dining out frequently may be detrimental to your health. Continue reading to find out how fast food affects your health.

Effect on the cardiovascular and digestive systems

With little to no fiber, most fast food items, including drinks and sides, are high in carbs.

These foods contain carbohydrates, which your digestive system breaks down and releases into your bloodstream as glucose (sugar). Your blood sugar rises as a result. In response to the spike in glucose, your pancreas releases insulin. Your body uses insulin to carry sugar to the cells that require it for energy. Your blood sugar levels return to normal when your body either consumes or stores the sugar.

Your body regulates this blood sugar process to a great extent. Your organs can normally withstand these spikes in sugar as long as you're in good health. However, eating a lot of carbohydrates often can cause your blood sugar to increase repeatedly. These insulin surges may eventually lead to a decline in your body's regular insulin response. This raises your risk of weight gain, type 2 diabetes, and insulin resistance.

Fat and sugar

A lot of fast food dishes have extra sugar. That translates to more calories without more nutrients. The American Heart Association recommends that adults limit their daily intake of added sugar to approximately 100 calories, or 6 teaspoons, for women and 150 calories, or 9 teaspoons, for men.

Just a few fast food beverages have more sugar in them than is advised daily. Coca-Cola has 9.75 teaspoons of sugar in a 12-ounce can. That amounts to 39 grams of sugar, 140 calories, and no other nutrients.

Trans-fat, a synthetic fat produced during food processing, is another component frequently found in fast food. It frequently appears in:

Fried pies Pastries

Pizza crust

Breakers

Cookie-based

Trans-fat in any proportion is unhealthy. Consuming meals that contain it raises your risk of heart disease and type 2 diabetes while lowering your HDL (good cholesterol) and raising your LDL (bad cholesterol).

Sodium

For some people, the combination of fat, sugar, and high sodium (salt) content makes fast food taste better. However, diets heavy in sodium can cause water retention, which is why eating fast food might make you feel swollen, bloated, or puffy.

A high-sodium diet poses additional risks to individuals with high blood pressure. Sodium can strain your heart and circulatory system and raise blood pressure.

According to one study, 90% of respondents misjudged the amount of salt in their fast food meals. 993 persons were polled for the study, and it was discovered that the participants' estimates of the sodium content were more than 1,000 mg off.

Remember that people should consume no more than 2,300 mg of sodium per day, according to the Food and Drug Administration (FDA). Restaurant meals and processed foods account for almost 70% of salt intake.

Effects on respiratory health

Weight gain may result from eating too many calories from fast food. Obesity may result from this. Breathlessness and other respiratory issues, such as asthma, are more likely to occur in obese people.

The excess weight can put strain on your heart and lungs, and even light exercise may cause symptoms to appear. Breathing problems could occur when you're exercising, walking, or climbing stairs.

Eating out might make keeping track of calories more difficult. Studies show that consumers frequently estimate menu items' caloric content incorrectly.

Effect on the central nervous system

Your brain and spinal cord make up your central nervous system. Eating fast food may also have an effect on these parts of your body.

According to a 2020 study, eating more fast food—and, surprisingly, salad—was associated with a worse short-term memory score in college students.

Effects on the reproductive system

The components in fast food and junk food may affect your ability to conceive. Processed food has been shown in one research to contain phthalates.

Phthalates are substances that can interfere with the physiological effects of hormones. High exposure to these substances may cause problems with reproduction, including problems with a fetus's development.

Effect on integumentary system (nails, skin, and hair)

Your skin's appearance may be affected by the meals you consume.

Though further research is required, a research analysis from 2021 indicated that meals high in fat, dairy, chocolate, and carbs and sugar with a high glycemic index were linked to acne. These items are frequently found in fast food.

On the other hand, the study indicated that consuming fatty acids (found in fish and olive oil), fruits, and vegetables helped prevent acne.

Effect on the skeletal structure (bones)

Acid reflux can be exacerbated by the carbohydrates and sugar found in processed and fast cuisine. Tooth enamel can be dissolved by certain acids. Cavities may form as a result of bacteria taking hold of your teeth as the enamel wears away. Complications with your muscle mass and bone density might also result from obesity. Particularly in older persons, obesity may result in poorer bone quality and an increased risk of bone fractures.

Maintaining a nutritious diet and regular exercise are crucial for building muscle, which supports your bones, and preventing bone loss.

Effect on psychological well-being

Fast food consumption can have an impact on both your physical and mental health.

According to a 2020 study, middle school children in China who ate fast food and sugary drinks had a higher risk of developing mental health problems.

According to research published in 2018, 14-year-old participants' body mass index (BMI) and inflammation were found to be greater when they had a Western diet heavy in red meat, takeaway, and refined foods. When they were 17 years old, this was linked to mental health problems and depression symptoms.

The social effects of fast food

Over one in five youngsters and over two out of every five adults in the United States are obese today. Fast food businesses' offerings might be a factor. According to one study, there was a considerable increase in portion sizes and caloric content in restaurant entrées and desserts between 1986 and 2016.

The increased frequency of eating out among Americans may have negative consequences for both the country's healthcare system and its citizens.

6 strategies to cut junk food out of your diet

Why does the issue of junk food concern nutrition experts? Excessive consumption might suppress your natural appetite and substitute unhealthy options with high-fat, high-salt, or high-sugar foods and beverages.

Snacks, meals, and reasonably priced beverages abound in our society. Frequently, more nutrient-dense foods like fruits, vegetables, whole grains, lean protein, and low-fat dairy are replaced by these excessively calorie-dense, high-calorie goods.

Foods with minimal nutritional value but wonderful flavors that appeal to our senses—such as smells, textures, and colors—overwhelm our bodies and minds. The following six suggestions can assist you in avoiding junk food and choosing healthy options:

1. Eat Frequently to Avoid Being Overly Hungry

Your stomach notifies your brain's reward system to react to any food cues it detects if you are overly hungry. Aim to adhere to a regular meal plan, avoid fad diets, and incorporate enough of fruits and vegetables along with healthful meals in your daily diet.

2. Start with a glass of water and stop drinking anything with added sugar

Drinks high in sugar, such as soda, energy drinks, sports drinks, and sweetened teas, might cause weight gain. We do not know the cause of this. One explanation for this could be that people drink somewhat less food when they drink a glass of regular cola than when they drink a zero-calorie glass of water or diet cola, which could lead the brain to misinterpret liquid calories.

3. Snack on nutrient-dense, low-calorie foods

Are you ever famished in between meals? Consider having some fresh fruit or vegetable sticks with hummus as a snack. Choose meals that you like that are low in fat, salt, and sugar and also low in calories. Choose meals you enjoy eating to prevent cravings for junk food.

Food taken at meals and in between, needs to satisfy our stomach and brain.

4. Recognize Your Sources of Stress

Observe the emotional cues that can cause you to seek appetizing junk food. Walk, talk to a friend, try meditation, or find another way to divert your attention. Stressful environments will make you need food, which will lead your blood sugar to spike and fall quickly, affecting your cardiovascular health and level of energy. Making healthy food and drink choices rather than calorie-dense ones will help you prepare ahead of time for how you will respond to these triggers. In order to keep our body healthy and balanced while under stress, we must drink plenty of water and eat a balanced diet.

6. Keep a positive attitude while acknowledging the drawbacks of marketing.

Junk food is enticing because of the clever marketing that it receives on television, the internet, and other media. Recognize that it can be challenging to substitute these high-calorie options with nutritious snacks and meals. Recall that most days, it is challenging for people to eat and drink healthful meals and beverages due to our current food environment. Make healthier meal choices and avoid junk food by starting small.

In summary, we are aware that junk food is enticing, reasonably priced, and easily accessible. Because of this, reducing our intake of junk food is difficult. On the other hand, there may be detrimental effects on our health if junk food starts to dominate our diets. Our diets should focus on high-fiber items such whole grains, fruits, and vegetables; meals with moderation in sugar and salt; and foods high in calcium and iron. Eating well contributes to the development of robust bodies and minds. Reducing consumption of junk food can be accomplished by governmental initiatives and health-promoting legislation, as well as individual dietary choices. Government assistance is required to restrict the advertising of junk food corporations to minors and to replace junk food outlets with healthier alternatives. Researchers can collaborate with young people to create solutions while concentrating on health promotion and education regarding healthy dietary options. Together, we can empower youth globally to make better eating choices that will benefit their immediate and long-term health.

The ideal diets for 5 prevalent medical conditions

You are aware that your general health and well-being are directly impacted by what you consume, and more often by what you don't. The answer to the question "What kind of diet should I be on?" could depend on a medical condition you now have. For certain medical problems, there are certain diets that can assist with symptom management, flare-up prevention, and treatment support.

The appropriate balance of meals can minimize symptoms produced by issues with the reproductive, cardiovascular, gastrointestinal, and endocrine systems, among other issues. Diet has a major role in improving many chronic health diseases.

When it comes to choosing the ideal diet, there is no one size fits all solution. various disorders require various diets. It may be worthwhile to change your diet and nutritional habits if any of the following apply to you in order to optimize your health.

IBS

Fatty liver

High blood pressure

PCOS

Overweight or obese

I.B.S

10 to 15 % of Americans suffer from the widespread gastrointestinal tract ailment known as irritable bowel syndrome, or IBS. It results in symptoms like:

Cramps in the abdomen

Swelling

Gas

Mucus In the stool

Alterations in the frequency and appearance of bowel movements

Some IBS sufferers experience diarrhea, while others may experience constipation and vice versa. The condition doesn't harm the intestines, although it can be uncomfortable.

Although the precise etiology of IBS is unknown, researchers have discovered that women are twice as likely as males to get the illness. The majority of IBS diagnoses occur in those under 45. Additionally, you run a higher risk if mental health problems or IBS run in your family.

IBS cannot be precisely tested. To rule out other problems, your healthcare professional could obtain X-rays, blood, and stool samples. In order to check for alterations or anomalies in your intestine, such as colitis, they could also recommend a colonoscopy.

You may experience intermittent symptoms from IBS for the remainder of your life. Even if there isn't a treatment for the illness, you can control it with food and medication. IBS is not caused by what you eat, however specific foods can occasionally trigger a flare-up.

The top 3 diets for IBS

So, when you have IBS, which foods are acceptable to eat and which ones should you avoid? While some people with IBS may have issues with particular foods, there is no one-size-fits-all IBS diet or solution.

1.The Low-FODMAP Diet

When treating food sensitivities and intolerances, many medical professionals will advise an elimination diet. One food at a time, you'll cut back on others until you identify the one that's giving you symptoms.

For IBS, a low-FODMAP diet is the typical elimination diet. Fermentable oligosaccharides, disaccharides, monosaccharides, and polyols is referred to as FODMAP. Some patients with IBS have cramps, diarrhea, constipation, stomach bloating, and gas after eating high-FODMAPS foods because their tiny intestines have difficulty absorbing these particular forms of carbohydrates.

A low-FODMAP diet entails giving up or reducing:

GOS and fructans are present in wheat, rye, onions, garlic, and legumes.

High fructose corn syrup, apples, and honey all contain fructose.

Goods containing the sweeteners sorbitol, mannitol, xylitol, and maltitol (which finish in -ol) The low-FODMAPS diet is intended to be short-term. For a few weeks, you will try it and see whether your symptoms go better. Once you're feeling better, you can gradually reintroduce foods high in FODMAPs into your diet. You can restrict or stay away from the foods that are triggering your IBS symptoms once you've identified them.

Working with a nutritionist or dietitian who has received training in the low-FODMAPS diet may be beneficial because this diet is quite complicated.

2. Diet without gluten

A gluten-free diet is another method for reducing the symptoms of IBS. Rye, barley, and wheat all contain gluten, a protein. It can be found in:

Pasta

Cereal

Grains

A lot of processed food

Although gluten-free diets are typically recommended for those with celiac disease, or gluten sensitivity, studies have shown that they can also help reduce symptoms in those with IBS.

3. Diet heavy in fiber. Increasing the amount of fiber in a person's diet can

help soften and facilitate the passage of stool, which in turn encourages more frequent bowel movements in those with IBS-C.

It is believed that soluble fiber, which is present in fruit, beans, and oat products, lessens the symptoms of IBS. While most Americans should strive for 25–35 grams of fiber per day, many only consume about 10-15 grams. Fiber-sensitive IBS patients should gradually increase their daily intake of it, starting at two to three grams.

Before your body is ready, consuming too much fiber might cause bloating and gas.

9 foods to avoid if you have IBS

Food triggers for IBS might vary from person to person, but some foods are more likely to produce issues than others. Your doctor may advise you to reduce or completely wipe out certain foods from your diet:

Carbonated drinks: These might exacerbate symptoms by causing gas and bloating.

Alcoholic drinks: As anyone who has experienced a hangover will attest, alcohol can have a negative internal impact. It may hasten the digestion process, making diarrhea worse.

Dairy: Some people may get cramps, diarrhea, constipation, stomach bloating, and gas due to the lactose included in milk and cheese. The intolerance to lactose may be associated to IBS.

Sugar: Fructose in particular can exacerbate the symptoms of IBS. IBS and sugar intolerance may be related.

Artificial sweeteners: Products like xylitol, sorbital, high fructose corn syrup, and others may have comparable effects on the digestive tract as sugar.

Processed foods: These items frequently have high levels of fat, sugar, and chemical additives, all of which might cause symptoms.

Like alcohol, caffeine accelerates the contraction of the intestines, called peristalsis, which exacerbates diarrhea.

Chemical additions: These have the potential to alter the gut microbiome and exacerbate symptoms of IBS.

Foods high in fat: For those with IBS, eating foods high in fat can slow down bowel motility and increase gas production.

Fatty liver

Fatty liver disease: what is it? It is a medical disorder where fat cells accumulate in the liver, as the name implies. There are two primary kinds: nonalcoholic (occurs even if you've never taken a drink) and alcohol-induced (produced by excessive alcohol consumption). Alcoholic fatty liver disease affects about 5% of people in the US. Moreover, nonalcoholic fatty liver disease (NAFLD), the most prevalent liver disease in children, affects about 200 million individuals worldwide. Nonalcoholic steato hepatitis (NASH) is the more severe kind, and it can lead to more serious illnesses such liver cancer and cirrhosis of the liver. Is having a fat liver harmful? While 1 in 5 people with fatty liver disease who drink excessively may get alcoholic hepatitis, most NASH and NAFLD patients won't have any serious problems. And it doesn't have to be a lifelong condition, which is wonderful news. Your greatest option if you're wondering how to reverse fatty liver disease is to make lifestyle adjustments including cutting alcohol, eating a fatty liver diet, and losing weight.

Although alcohol intake is frequently the cause of fatty liver disease, this is not always the case. Fatty liver disease is one of the main causes of liver failure.

Regardless of the reason, you can reduce the amount of fat deposits in your liver by following a low-calorie, low-fat diet and decreasing weight. Consuming a diet high in leafy greens, whole grains, nuts, seeds, and healthy fats can help reduce the buildup of fat in the body. Eat fish and meat that is lean rather than greasy. Last but not least, abstain from alcohol but not caffeine, as some research indicates that consuming caffeine may lower the incidence of liver cirrhosis and fibrosis.

Making deliberate and long-lasting dietary modifications is crucial for treating fatty liver disease, as opposed to merely avoiding or including certain foods sometimes.

What foods are beneficial for liver repair? The most essential thing about these adjustments is that they should be sustainable. The ideal NAFLD and NASH diets often consist of:

Sufficient fiber

An abundance of nuts, fruits, and veggies

Whole grains

Very little animal-derived saturated fat

Extremely little sugar and salt

Absent alcohol

8 foods to eat

In particular, experts advise eating these foods to maintain a healthy liver:

Low-fat dairy products or almond milk: People with fatty liver disease, both adults and children, should be mindful of their calcium intake. Furthermore, individuals with advanced liver illness may experience early osteopenia and osteoporosis as well as multiple nutritional issues. It is not always the case that fatty liver disease reduces the absorption of calcium. Calcium is just necessary for everyone. You can either take calcium and vitamin D supplements (the recommended dosage for calcium is 1,000–1,200 mg and for vitamin D is

2,000–5,000 IU if you are deficient) or consume up to three glasses of each type of milk each day.

Coffee: Research has revealed that coffee, when consumed without additional sugar or creamers, is now one of the best treatments to treat fatty liver. Coffee seems to lessen the gut's permeability, which makes it harder for people to absorb lipids. The full answer to this query is yet unknown, though, as this is currently being looked at. However, a growing body of research suggests that coffee can help prevent fatty liver disease. It may be advised to have multiple cups of coffee, depending on the patient.

Vitamin E-rich foods: Vitamin E-rich foods, such as red bell peppers, spinach, peanuts, and pecans, are a fantastic complement to diets for those with fatty livers. Further research is necessary, although one study finds that those with NAFLD or NASH can see a slight improvement with the vitamin. A daily dose of 400–800 IU is advised.

Water: Experts advised using water instead of sugary and calorie-dense beverages whenever feasible. In order to prevent dehydration and its detrimental effects on the liver, the average person should drink half an ounce to an ounce of water for every pound of body weight each day, assuming they do not have any medical problems that would limit their consumption of fluids.

Olive oil: Certain oils, like avocado and olive oils, can supply good fats. They lower the levels of liver enzymes and aid in satiety. Other oils high in monounsaturated fats include safflower, canola, sesame, peanut, and sunflower oils.

Flax and chia seeds: Omega-3 acids can be found in plants like flax and chia seeds. Since these acids may lower the amount of fat in the liver, they are beneficial for fatty livers that are not caused by alcohol or drugs.

Garlic: According to one study, increasing your intake of garlic over a 15-week period resulted in decreased body fat mass in persons with NAFLD as well as reduced liver fat and avoided the disease's progression. The study focused on garlic powder, but other forms of the herb also perform well.

Soy: According to some research, soy-based items like tofu and soy milk may help with fatty liver. According to one study, studies have indicated improvements in the metabolic parameters of NAFLD patients.

8 foods to stay away from

Generally speaking, the foods to stay away from are those that can cause blood sugar spikes or weight gain, like:

Sugars and carbs are the enemies of the liver; these include juice, soda, sugary drinks, and refined carbohydrates like white bread.

Diet beverages with little calories: Substitutes for sugar may potentially worsen liver disease.

Foods heavier in saturated fat, such as butter and ghee, have been linked to elevated triglycerides in the liver.

Sweet baked products and desserts, such as pies, cakes, pastries, ice cream, and so on: If you are trying to reverse fatty liver disease, these kinds of sugary carbohydrates will not help your cause.

Bacon, sausage, cured meats, and other high-fat meat products are not advised because they contain a lot of saturated fat.

Alcohol: Consuming alcohol can only worsen liver damage if you already have fatty liver disease, which is caused by heavy drinking. It's acceptable for people with NAFLD to occasionally drink alcohol, such as a glass of wine.

Salty foods: According to some research, eating salt may exacerbate NAFLD for two reasons. It usually goes well with foods that are heavier in fat and calories, like some of the items on this list. It can also cause the renin-angiotensin system to become dysregulated, which increases your chance of developing fatty liver.

Fried foods: Contrary to professional recommendations to adhere to a more calorie-restricted diet, fried meals such as French fries and onion rings are frequently rich in calories.

High blood pressure

The enigmatic reason of high blood pressure is common. A number of factors, including age, stress levels, lifestyle choices, family history, and medical issues, are linked to it. What is less ambiguous? The remedies for this widespread ailment. If you have been diagnosed with hypertension, there are proven ways to lower your blood pressure levels. Blood pressure can be managed by consuming certain foods and avoiding others.

Risk factors for hypertension include heavy metal poisoning, using some birth control pills, smoking, drinking alcohol, eating an unhealthy diet high in sodium, being obese, and experiencing mental stress.

Your doctor might advise you to make lifestyle adjustments if you have hypertension, like eating a healthy diet with less salt and getting frequent exercise. By lowering your blood pressure, these changes may help lessen your risk of heart disease and other linked health problems.

DASH eating plan

Are you unsure about what to eat to bring down your blood pressure? Dietary approaches to stop hypertension, or DASH diet, is one of the best dietary strategies for lowering blood pressure. The DASH diet is low in foods high in saturated fats, high in fruits, vegetables, and whole grains, and low in sodium (less than 2300 mg daily).

Foods to consume

A balanced diet that includes all of the recommended foods can help lower blood pressure, even though there isn't one particular meal that can do so. Grain, fruit, vegetable, and legume fiber are good foods for high blood pressure.

Minerals from whole grains, such as magnesium, combine with calcium from low-fat dairy to enhance your health. Vegetables and fruits contain potassium. Potassium eases the strain in your blood vessels and lessens the effects of salt.

The following foods are high in potassium and are among the best for lowering blood pressure: avocados, carrots, melons (cantaloupe or honeydew), dairy products (fat-free or low-fat), spinach, greens, fish (tuna and halibut), legumes, mushrooms, orange juice, potatoes, prunes, and dates, raisins and dates, tomatoes, and olives.

Foods to avoid

It is best to stay away from highly processed foods, saturated fats, salt, fried foods, and excessive alcohol consumption. It is also detrimental to your blood pressure to consume more calories than you should every day. A calorie surplus leads to weight growth.

Blood pressure is increased by excess weight.

Blood pressure can also rise with diets heavy in salt, which is included in a lot of cured or smoked foods and sauces. Avoid eating these meals since they may cause your blood pressure to rise:

Processed meats like hot dogs and bacon

Food items in cans with preservatives

Foods high in salt, including potato chips and pickles

Fried dishes like chicken strips and French fries

Red meat in particular is high in fat.

Margarine and vegetable oil, which are heavy in trans-fat

Table Liquid

Grapes

Note: Certain blood pressure drugs may have harmful interactions with grapefruit and grapefruit juice. Before making any dietary changes, speak with a doctor or nutritionist about potential drug interactions and food interactions.

In general, follow a low-sodium diet that includes lean meat and fewer added sugars to boost your heart health. To cut back on sodium intake, read food labels and steer clear of items high in sugar, such as fruit juices and some salad dressings.

PCOS

Between 6% and 12% of American women who are of reproductive age suffer from polycystic ovarian syndrome, or PCOS. It results in an imbalance of hormones, mainly an increase in androgen (male hormones), which causes thinning hair, excessive facial and body hair growth, acne, irregular periods, and even infertility. Insulin resistance and weight gain are linked to the disorder.

Modifications to diet and lifestyle may help control body weight and lower insulin resistance, which may lessen the severity of other symptoms. But which diet plan, if you have PCOS, should you pick among the plethora of options available? The optimal diet for someone with PCOS varies based on their symptoms. Eating practices that reduce the risk of related illnesses, control blood sugar, reduce insulin resistance, and help manage weight (if necessary) should ideally be followed. The ideal diet is one that you can stick to over time, is realistic and manageable, doesn't feel restrictive, and balances your intake of carbs, fats, proteins, and fiber-rich foods to keep your blood sugar steady all day.

8 foods to eat

1. Vegetables and fruits

Eat less fruit that has a high glycemic index, like watermelon. To begin with, here are some excellent fruits and vegetables:

Sprouts

Lettuce

Green beans

Onion

Fruits

Raspberries

Banana

It's also crucial to select a rainbow of fruits and veggies.

2. Seeds and nuts

These are an excellent source of anti-inflammatory compounds, healthy fats like omega-3s, and protein. This is beneficial for PCOS sufferers since they frequently have a low-grade inflammation that triggers the production of androgen in the ovaries. Heart and blood vascular issues may result from this. Try the following nuts and seeds:

Almonds

Cashews

Walnuts

Sesame

Sunflower

Pumpkin

Flax (use pre-ground or freshly ground flax seeds instead of whole ones)

Chia

Nuts and seeds are great as a snack on their own, added to meals (like oatmeal), sprinkled over salads, or mixed into smoothies.

3. Fish rich in omega-3 fatty acids

People with PCOS can benefit from this essential healthy fat because it can help with cholesterol and insulin resistance. Numerous fish species contain omega-3 fatty acids, such as:

Salmon

Mackerel

Shrimp

Herring

Oysters

Sardines

Anchovies

Caviar

4. Whole wheat

Compared to processed grains, whole grains include more fiber and are an excellent source of protein. For those with PCOS, high-fiber diets are crucial because they reduce the risk of blood sugar rises, which increase the amount of insulin released into the system. Those who are sensitive to insulin may experience issues including trouble losing weight due to high insulin levels. Among the nutritious whole grains are the following:

Whole oats

Whole wheat

Barley whole grain

Millet

Quinoa

Popcorn

Whole wheat bread

Whole-wheat spaghetti

Additionally, whole grains prolong feelings of fullness, reducing the likelihood of overindulging.

5. Plant-based and lean proteins

Not all proteins are created equal, but they do aid in encouraging healthy muscle growth, lowering blood sugar surges, and increasing feelings of satisfaction. Choose fish, poultry, and other non-red meats more frequently if you're looking for meatless protein. Because lean protein has fewer calories while providing the same quantity of protein, it is preferable to fatty meat. It's also possible to have enough protein without consuming meat. Among the excellent plant-based proteins are:

Tofu

Chickpeas

Lentils

Hempseed

Quinoa

Soybeans

You probably don't need as much protein as you would assume. A deck of cards is around the size of a meal of protein.

6. Full-fat dairy products and substitutes

For those with PCOS, full-fat dairy is advised over low- or no-fat dairy products since it may enhance fertility. Here are a few instances of dairy products that are advised:

Whole milk

Cheese

Plain Greek yogurt

Almond milk, oat milk, and fortified soy milk are some options if you don't eat dairy.

7. Spices

People with PCOS may be able to reduce inflammation and lose weight by following an anti-inflammatory diet. The following are a few spices that may have anti-inflammatory qualities: Ginger, Cinnamon, Turmeric, Cayenne, and Garlic

8. Adequate fats

An adequate diet must include fats. Fats aid in the absorption of vitamins since many vitamins are fat-soluble. Additionally, they minimize or avoid blood sugar surges, which are detrimental to PCOS patients. Particularly for those with PCOS who are at risk of heart disease, it is crucial to pick healthy fats over saturated or trans fats, such as hydrogenated oils, and to take them in moderation. Seek out:

Extra virgin olive oil

Avocado oil

Walnut oil

Flaxseed oil

Foods to stay away from if you have PCOS

With the exception of zero- or low-calorie sweeteners, which she advises against using because they have been shown to enhance sugar cravings and are associated with weight gain, people with PCOS shouldn't feel as though they must fully eliminate any one food unless they are allergic, sensitive, or intolerant to anything.

Instead, individuals with PCOS should consider their diet as a whole and concentrate on assembling a well-balanced diet of wholesome foods.

Certain foods might cause blood sugar increases or increase insulin levels in those who have PCOS. While certain foods are permitted, one should limit them.

1. Refined sweets and simple carbs

Baked products made mostly of simple carbohydrates, such cakes, cookies, pastries, etc. Soft drinks, a lot of juices, white bread, rice, pasta, and similar meals have a high glycemic index, which means that they enter cells fast and release more insulin into the bloodstream. This leads to an increase in blood sugar levels and exacerbates insulin resistance.

2. Foods that are processed

Just as simple carbs can cause insulin resistance, so too can highly processed meals. They frequently lack the fiber found in raw meals and have extra sugar and salt. For example, the fiber in an entire apple helps to reduce the surge in blood sugar. Much of the fiber is processed out by applesauce, which speeds up the body's absorption of the sugar. After additional processing, apple juice causes a sudden surge in blood sugar. This also applies to many processed meals, including processed canned noodles as opposed to whole grain al dente pasta.

3. Trans-fats and saturated fats

An elevated risk of cardiovascular illness exists in those with PCOS. Use of saturated fat should be limited, and a lot of medical professionals advise against consuming trans-fats at all. Processed foods contain these fats, which can reduce the nutritional value of nutritious foods. Butter-cooked eggs and veggies are not as healthful as, say, poached eggs and steamed veggies.

Overweight or obese

There is disagreement on the relationship between body mass index (BMI) and health. The BMI, which has been in use for than 200 years, determines whether your current size is optimum for you based on your height and weight. BMI values are derived from statistics and can be inaccurate, particularly for older people, athletes, and pregnant women. This is because weight from muscle mass is not included in the calculations. On the other hand, those with greater BMIs are more susceptible to a number of chronic illnesses, including Arthritis, sleep apnea, diabetes, high blood pressure, heart disease, and liver damage.

At various times throughout your life, your BMI might start to trend toward being overweight or obese. Your doctor might then advise you to lose weight for health-related reasons. Remaining at a healthy weight helps improve blood pressure management and lessen the strain on your circulatory system, among other health benefits. Keep reading to discover healthy and effective weight loss methods if you're trying to shed a few pounds.

5 meals to eat

There are plenty of options available to you if you wish to include healthful foods in your diet that have been linked to weight loss. You should consume fat, protein, and carbohydrates in moderation while preserving a calorie deficit. This often entails introducing whole grains, low-fat dairy, non-starchy vegetables, fruits, lean proteins, healthy fats, and whole grains into your diet. These six foods have been shown to help with weight loss, so you might want to give them some thought.

First, olive oil

Given that olive oil is high in calories, you probably do not associate it with diet foods. However, studies have shown that olive oil helps people lose weight. In fact, the well-known Mediterranean diet encourages people to use olive oil as their primary fat source. Olive oil is a healthy fat, and according to one study, people who use it are less likely to be obese. Just remember to use it sparingly because, although healthful, it is a high-fat condiment.

Second, Lean meats

Since the body needs protein to create muscle, it should be a part of every diet. Select lean meats instead of fatty red meat cuts when choosing proteins because they are heart-healthy and lower in fat. What precisely are lean meats then? The American Heart Association states that fish, skinless chicken, and the leanest cuts of red meat are the best sources of animal protein. In addition to being low in calories, lean meats are an excellent source of zinc, iron, B vitamins, and fatty acids.

Third, Legumes

Though they are delicious for everyone, beans are a fantastic natural plant-based source of protein for vegetarians and vegans. Beans, peas, lentils, soybeans, and peanuts are examples of legumes. Legumes and weight loss has been the subject of several research, the majority of which found beneficial relationships. According to a comprehensive assessment of the literature, people who combine beans with a low-calorie diet may be more successful in losing weight than those who follow a traditional low-calorie diet without them. Legumes have a lot of fiber as well. Fiber improves blood sugar regulation and helps you feel fuller for longer periods of time.

Forth, Whole grain

Most certainly, you've heard that giving up carbohydrates will help you lose weight. However, certain carbs are beneficial to you! Eating whole grains, such brown rice, oats, and whole-grain bread or pasta, is the greatest way to get carbohydrates. According to a comprehensive research published in 2020, people who ate three servings of whole grains a day on average had lower BMIs. In contrast to those who consumed fewer whole grains, study participants who consumed more whole grains also had better lifestyles and engaged in greater physical activity.

Fifth, Broth-based soups

Pay attention to foods that are low in calories, high in nutrients, and large in volume. Soups with a broth basis are one food item that satisfies all three criteria. Foods rich in volume fill you up, and foods high in nutrients, such as fiber, phytonutrients, and micronutrients, promote health and wellness. Soups with broth base are low in calories and can help you lose weight. Just be careful that these are broth-based soups that are thin rather than thick and creamy soups, which can have more calories.

4 foods to stay away from

Which foods are you not supposed to eat when on a diet? It shouldn't be necessary for most people to completely eliminate any foods. You can incorporate a dish that you truly appreciate into your diet. Foods that are extremely refined, heavy in sugar and fat, and lack true nutritional value should be consumed in moderation. These foods raise blood sugar and cholesterol levels in addition to causing weight gain. They can soon surpass your daily calorie intake and be detrimental to your health. Therefore, it's advisable to limit the foods on this list when making dietary modifications for weight loss, even though you can enjoy them in moderation.

1. Sweetened beverage

Sweetened coffee drinks and sodas are examples of sugary beverages that are empty calories. In other words, you won't feel full after drinking them all day. After a meal, satiety is the sensation of fullness. A study conducted in 2011 concluded that there is "accumulating evidence suggesting that liquid carbohydrates generally produce less satiety than solid forms." With 140 calories in a single can, Coca-Cola may build up quickly over time. If your goal is to lose weight, try selecting drinks without added sugar and consuming fewer of them.

2. Alcohol

Liquor contains empty calories that don't make you feel full, much like sugary drinks do. Studies have shown that drinking alcohol can lead to an increased risk of weight gain. That might, however, vary depending on your preference for and volume of alcohol consumption. According to a systematic analysis, people who drink heavily are more likely to gain weight, whereas people who drink light to moderately—especially wine—are more likely to stay underweight. This research found that while the occasional glass of wine is probably not going to make you gain weight, drinking spirits is likely to make you gain weight.

3. Sugary treats

Who doesn't enjoy cookies, cakes, and donuts? These sweet treats are difficult to resist. In fact, research has shown that the brain's reward system responds to excessively sugary foods in the same manner that it does to drugs and gambling. Treats are empty calories with no nutritious benefit, so you should only have them occasionally. They can raise insulin and blood sugar levels in addition to causing weight gain.

4. Granola bar

It's common to see granola bars and energy bars promoted as excellent providers of fiber, protein, and daily nutrients. However, did you realize that some of these bars have sugar content comparable to that of a candy bar? If you look at the label the next time you're about to buy a bar at the store, you might be astonished to see how much sugar is added. Have a handful of nuts, some fresh fruit, or some yogurt without added sugar as a quick snack on the run.

Additional useful resources for weight loss:

Exercise

Sufficient sleep

- Appropriate intake of water

- Changes in medication

CONCLUSION

There will always be a dispute between junk food and nutritious food, but when it comes to enhancing overall health and lowering the risk of chronic illnesses, it is obvious that healthy food wins. But it's crucial to keep in mind that when it comes to your nutrition, moderation and balance are essential. While the occasional indulgence in junk food is OK, it's crucial to make healthy decisions the majority of the time. You can use the knowledge in this book as a reference to help you make wise eating choices, and always remember to put your health first.